What you really need to know about

HIGH BLOOD PRESSURE

Dr Robert Buckman
with Patsy Westcott

Introduced by John Cleese

MARSHALL PUBLISHING • LONDON

A Marshall Edition
Conceived by Marshall Editions
The Orangery
161 New Bond Street
London W1Y 9PA
Edited and designed by Axis Design, 8 Accommodation Road, London NW11 8ED

First published in the UK in 1999 by
Marshall Publishing Ltd
Copyright © 1999 Marshall Editions Developments Ltd

ISBN: 1 84028 248 7

Originated in Italy by Articolor
Printed in and bound in Italy by New Interlitho

Managing Editor For Axis Design Jo Wells
Project Editor Theresa Reynolds
Indexer Susan Bosanko
Art Editor Siân Keogh
Illustrator Kuo Kang Chen
Photographer David Jordan
Managing Editor Anne Yelland
Managing Art Editor Helen Spencer
Editorial Director Ellen Dupont
Art Director Dave Goodman
Editorial Coordinator Becca Clunes
Production Nikki Ingram, Anna Pauletti
DTP Mike Grigoletti

The consultant for this book, Dr. Michael Schachter, BSc, MB, BS, MRCP, is Senior Lecturer
in Clinical Pharmacology at Imperial College School of Medicine, London, and Honorary
Consultant Physician at St Mary's Hospital, London. Dr. Schachter specializes in basic and
clinical research in cardiovascular therapeutics.

Contents

Foreword

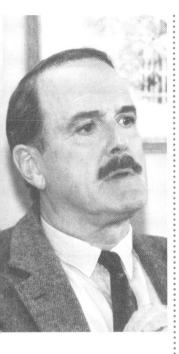

Most of you know me best as someone who makes people laugh.

But for 30 years I have also been involved with communicating information. And one particular area in which communication often breaks down is the doctor/patient relationship. We have all come across doctors who fail to communicate clearly, using complex medical terms when a simple explanation would do, and dismiss us with a "come back in a month if you still feel unwell". Fortunately, I met Dr Robert Buckman.

Rob is one of North America's leading experts on cancer, but far more importantly he is a doctor who believes that hiding behind medical jargon is unhelpful and unprofessional. He wants his patients to understand what is wrong with them, and spends many hours with them—and their families and close friends—making sure they understand everything. Together we created a series of videos, with the jargon-free title *Videos for Patients*. Their success has prompted us to write books that explore medical conditions in the same clear, simple terms.

This book is one of a series that will tell you all you need to know about your condition. It assumes nothing. If you have a helpful, honest, communicative doctor, you will find here the extra information that he or she simply may not have time to tell you. If you are less fortunate, this book will help to give you a much clearer picture of your situation.

More importantly—and this was a major factor in the success of the videos—you can access the information here again and again. Turn back, read over, until you really know what your doctor's diagnosis means.

In addition, because in the middle of a consultation, you may not think of everything you would like to ask your doctor, you can also use the book to help you formulate the questions you would like to discuss with him or her.

John Cleese

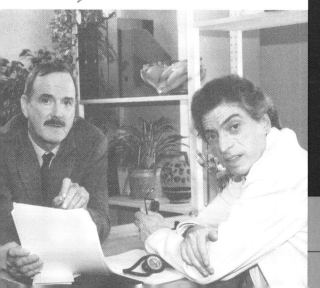

Introduction

High blood pressure is one of the most common conditions in the Western world. It is thought that one adult in four has moderately raised blood pressure and around one in 13 has it severely.

Although many people imagine high blood pressure to be a mild condition, left untreated it can lead to a number of serious medical problems. Research has shown that failure to control raised blood pressure is the leading cause of stroke. It also puts you at risk of angina or heart attack, heart failure and kidney damage. In those people who have diabetes, it can be responsible for serious eyesight problems which may result in blindness.

Your BP, as it is known in the medical profession, is the force exerted on the walls of the arteries as your heart pumps blood through the vast circulatory network of arteries, veins and millions of capillaries.

In a healthy body the blood vessel walls are flexible and nothing impedes the blood flow as it constantly moves around the body delivering nutrient-rich oxygen to all the cells and carrying away the waste products to be eliminated. When the walls are adversely affected and lose their elasticity, the blood supply is not as it should be and the heart has to work harder to make it reach every part of the body.

Be aware

The trouble is that you won't necessarily know this as an increase in blood pressure causes no symptoms. You might think you'd get headaches or nosebleeds, but it isn't so. This is why it is vitally important for everyone to know what their blood pressure is by having it checked regularly so that, if it is raised, it can be medically treated with blood-pressure-lowering drugs.

Taking control

As research into heart and kidney disease has brought greater understanding of the importance of blood pressure, more is being done today to treat hypertension. You can be assured that if you have high blood pressure there are many simple, effective treatments that can be tailored to you as an individual.

As we all learn more about the effect of lifestyle on health, people with high blood pressure have a range of practical self-help steps they can take. The simplest rules are paying attention to what you eat and drink, quitting smoking, becoming more active and avoiding stress. In mild cases these measures may even lower your blood pressure without the need for medication. Even if you do need blood pressure treatment, taking such steps can help increase the efficiency of treatment and give you a valuable sense of control.

Entering a partnership

Although it may be alarming to discover that you have high blood pressure, with treatment you have every chance of reducing it and increasing your chances of living a long, healthy life.

This book will tell you all you need to know about your blood pressure, how to find out if it is raised and what can be done about it if you have a problem. With the information available in these pages you are able to enter a partnership with your doctor so you will know what questions to ask and when to ask them. A diagnosis of hypertension is a warning sign that you need to play a greater part in your own health to prevent the development of much more serious problems. This book will help you do just that.

Chapter

1

SYMPTOMS & DIAGNOSIS

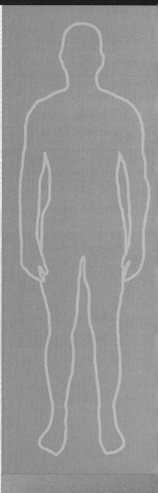

How the heart works

Your heart pumps blood through your blood vessels to supply every cell of your body with oxygen (from the lungs) and nutrients. With each beat your heart contracts, squeezing blood into the arteries and pumping it around your body. Blood is returned to the heart through the veins. The walls of the arteries are elastic, so they stretch slightly with each heartbeat to accommodate the surge of blood.

Tremendous force is needed to pump blood out of your heart and around your body. If you have high blood pressure the stress on the arteries is intense. As a result the smooth lining of the arteries becomes rough and their walls become thicker. Over time, this causes the arteries to narrow and become less elastic, a process known as arteriosclerosis or hardening of the arteries.

HOW BLOOD FLOWS AROUND THE BODY

Blood is pumped from the heart into the lungs where oxygen is added to it (this is called oxygenation). The oxygen-rich blood then returns to the heart, from where it is pumped to the brain and around the rest of the body, supplying oxygen to all of the cells. It returns, deoxygenated, to the heart, where the cycle begins again.

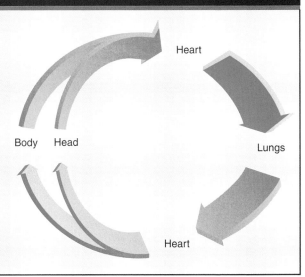

Heart

Lungs

Body   Head

Heart

10

ANGIOTENSIN

A hormone normally present in the body that acts on the blood vessels and causes them to narrow.

ARTERIOLE

A medium-sized blood vessel that branches off an artery.

ARTERIOSCLEROSIS

Hardening and narrowing of the arteries. Can be a major factor in raising blood pressure above the norm.

RENIN

A hormone produced by the kidneys.

How blood pressure is regulated

Blood pressure is regulated by both the brain and the kidneys. The area of your brain that controls circulation receives messages about the level of blood pressure from pressure-sensitive nerves in the arteries. It responds by instructing smaller blood vessels called arterioles to narrow or widen as necessary. This alters the pressure in the arteries.

Blood pressure is also partly regulated by a hormone, called renin, produced by the kidneys. The production of renin causes the release of another blood chemical, angiotensin, which narrows the arterioles and raises blood pressure. Angiotensin also causes the adrenal gland to release a hormone which makes your kidneys retain too much salt. Salt increases the volume of blood in circulation, which causes blood pressure to rise.

How the heart works

What is blood pressure?

The heart pumps blood around the body through large blood vessels known as arteries, supplying your body and brain with oxygen and essential nutrients. The pressure of the blood travelling in the arteries is determined by how hard the heart works and the health of your blood vessels. High blood pressure, or hypertension as it is known medically, is when this pressure becomes too high.

What is normal?

It may sound odd, but "normal" blood pressure varies a lot. It varies from one person to the next, and in any individual it rises and falls naturally during the course of each day, depending on the workload of the heart. What is more, everyone's blood pressure tends to rise slightly with age. Because of these differences, there is no set point at which high blood pressure is diagnosed. It depends on an individual's age and lifestyle.

HOW BLOOD PRESSURE CHANGES THOUGH A DAY

FOR MEN AND WOMEN

WHEN IT IS LOWER

◆ At night

◆ When you are relaxing

◆ When you are asleep

◆ When listening to quiet music.

WHEN IT IS HIGHER

◆ During the day

◆ With exercise or exertion

◆ While smoking a cigarette

◆ If anxious, stressed or excited

◆ In cold weather.

LOW BLOOD PRESSURE

Low blood pressure, or hypotension as it is known, is not usually a medical problem. In fact, by and large if your blood pressure is low you are more likely to live a long, healthy life. Shock caused by a heart attack or heavy blood loss after an accident can cause a sudden and sometimes dangerous fall in blood pressure. In such cases, fainting may occur because the heart cannot sustain the blood supply to the brain; however, once the person is horizontal, blood flows back to the brain and consciousness returns. Very occasionally, abnormally low blood pressure is a symptom of an illness that needs treatment.

In a normal, healthy young adult the average blood pressure measurement is around 120/80 (for an explanation of how blood pressure is measured, see p.14). Ideally, your blood pressure should stay below 140/85. If, however, your blood pressure is consistently higher than this, and certainly if it rises above 160/90, you will need medical treatment.

Is high blood pressure a problem?

High blood pressure is not an illness in itself. In fact, most people who have it feel perfectly well and do not experience any symptoms. However it is important that it is treated, because if it stays raised for any length of time it can damage the blood vessels and lead to serious health problems including eye problems, hardening of the arteries (arteriosclerosis), heart attack, stroke, heart failure and kidney failure (see p. 24).

YOU REALLY NEED TO KNOW

◆ High blood pressure can lead to stroke, hardened arteries, heart attack, heart failure and kidney failure.

◆ If your blood pressure is consistently raised you will probably need medical treatment.

◆ Only in rare cases does low blood pressure require treatment.

What is blood pressure?

Measuring blood pressure

DOs AND DON'Ts

✓ It's easier to take your BP if you wear a sleeveless top or one with loose fitting sleeves that can be rolled up.

✓ Try to relax your arm and breathe evenly when the nurse or doctor wraps the cuff around your arm.

✗ Don't drink tea, coffee or cola type drinks before having your blood pressure taken.

✗ Don't smoke a cigarette or use a nicotine replacement patch one or two hours before the BP's measured.

There are high-tech machines available for measuring blood pressure, but it is most common for doctors and nurses to use a device called a sphygmomanometer which is easier to use than it is to pronounce. It consists of a pump, an inflatable arm cuff and a column of mercury in a glass tube. The pressure in the cuff causes the mercury column to rise up the tube: the height of the

HAVING YOUR BLOOD PRESSURE TAKEN

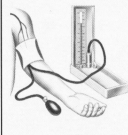

1 The cuff is placed around your upper arm and pumped up by the doctor or nurse, temporarily cutting off the blood flow. As a result your pulse can no longer be heard through a stethoscope placed against your arm.

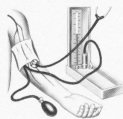

2 As the cuff pressure is slowly released blood flow is restored and the doctor or nurse listens for a thumping noise as your heart contracts. This is the first measurement, the systolic.

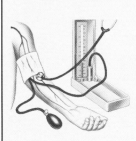

3 As your heart relaxes between beats, the mercury column drops as the sound of blood flow becomes less distinct. When it disappears, the second measurement, the diastolic, is recorded.

BLOOD PRESSURE ON THE MOVE

Portable devices can be used to measure your blood pressure as you go about your daily activities. A printout tells your doctor your average blood pressure over the course of the day. This is known as ambulatory blood pressure monitoring (ABPM). It gives a more realistic idea of your blood pressure over time and often produces a lower reading than one-off readings taken by the doctor.

column can be read in millimetres from the numbers printed on the tube. This is why blood pressure measurements are expressed in millimetres of mercury.

With each heartbeat, a pulse (surge) of blood is created in the arteries. The doctor or nurse can hear this pulse by placing a stethoscope on the brachial artery which runs through your arm. This one is used because it is one of the major arteries branching from the aorta, the main artery leading from your heart; and also, being in the forearm, is easily accessible which means you don't have to get undressed.

The person taking your blood pressure listens for your pulse and notes the measurement at the point when your heart contracts and when it relaxes (see box left).

Sometimes the doctor may take two readings of your blood pressure: one while you are seated and another when you are standing. This is because blood pressure sometimes dips when you stand up (especially in older people). If your blood pressure is raised, the doctor may measure it a few times during your visit to the surgery to get an average reading.

YOU REALLY NEED TO KNOW

◆ Cutting off the blood flow with the inflatable cuff for such a short time isn't harmful.

◆ The doctor or nurse listens for the sound of your pulse in the main artery running through your arm.

◆ There are two measurements taken—one when the pulse begins again (the higher) and another when it fades or disappears (the lower).

◆ If the doctor thinks the readings taken at the surgery were too high you may be asked to use a portable device to check your BP at frequent intervals as you go about your everyday life.

Measuring blood pressure

Blood pressure readings

KNOW THE TERMS

✓ The actual point in the heartbeat cycle when the heart contracts is known as a systole.

✓ The point in the cycle when the heart relaxes is called the diastole.

✓ Hypertension is raised blood pressure. Hypotension is below "normal" blood pressure.

A blood pressure reading consists of two figures, written as 120/80 and read as "120 over 80". The upper figure is the measurement taken when your heart is contracting and is known as the systolic pressure. The lower figure is the one taken when your heart relaxes, and is known as the diastolic pressure.

Systolic pressure

The pressure in your blood vessels is at its peak when your heart contracts to squeeze blood into the arteries. This systolic pressure, measured when the doctor or nurse first hears the sound of your heartbeat, reflects the work of your heart and can vary a lot depending on what you are doing.

In a healthy person the systolic pressure is normally between 120 and 140 millimetres of mercury, written as 120 or 140mm Hg (the chemical name for mercury).

Diastolic pressure

The pressure in your blood vessels is at its lowest when your heart relaxes and fills with blood. This is known as the diastolic blood pressure, which the doctor or nurse

ISOLATED SYSTOLIC HYPERTENSION

Sometimes the diastolic blood pressure is normal but the systolic blood pressure is raised. Doctors call this isolated systolic hypertension (ISH). You are mostly likely to have it if you are over 65 and if you do the doctor will want to prescribe treatment as you could be at high risk of developing heart disease or having a stroke.

records at the last sound of your heart beating. In a healthy person the diastolic pressure is around 80mm Hg. In general doctors prefer it not to go above 85, but 90 might be acceptable in some instances.

What the doctor is looking for

High blood pressure is diagnosed by looking at both the systolic and diastolic blood pressure. Usually if the systolic pressure is raised the diastolic pressure is too, and vice versa.

It used to be believed that raised diastolic pressure was more important than raised systolic pressure, because it is a sign that the medium-sized or small arteries have become stiff and narrowed. Research has now shown, however, that if you are over 40 a raised systolic pressure, which indicates how hard your heart is having to work, is also significant—especially in predicting whether you will develop heart disease.

Defining high blood pressure

There is no set measurement at which high blood pressure is treated. You may have borderline hypertension at 160/90 and treatment may depend on whether you have any other medical problems.

Your blood pressure tends to be defined as high if any of the following apply:

◆ the systolic pressure is 140 or higher.
◆ the diastolic is 90 or higher.
◆ both systolic and diastolic pressure are high.

The doctor will usually want to take measures to reduce your blood pressure to the ideal target of 140/85 if you are otherwise well, or to a lower 130/80 if you have type 2 (late onset) diabetes.

Blood pressure readings

Self monitoring

DOs AND DON'Ts

Do consult your doctor before buying a self-monitoring device.

Do make sure you are using a self-monitoring device correctly.

Do not worry about a single high blood pressure reading— this can happen for all sorts of reasons.

Occasionally the doctor might suggest that you monitor your own blood pressure at home to provide information on how you are responding to medication, especially when it is first prescribed. It can also help the doctor to ascertain whether blood pressure lies behind other symptoms, such as light headedness. Self-monitoring can be especially useful if you need to have your blood pressure checked one or more times a day, or to keep an eye on it over a period of time.

Self-monitoring devices

You can buy electronic, non-mercury automatic or semi-automatic machines to take your blood pressure at home. Some, like the sphygmomanometer used at the doctor's surgery, measure the pressure in the brachial artery in your arm. Others measure the pressure by monitoring the pulse at your wrist (though this is not regarded as very reliable) or your finger.

Not all home monitoring devices are equally reliable. Seek your doctor's advice before buying one.

Using a self-monitoring device

If you do decide to use a self-monitoring device, follow the instructions carefully and ask your doctor or nurse for help if you are in any doubt about how to use it. Finally, remember that a single high blood-pressure reading is unimportant. What matters is if your blood pressure is continually raised over a period of time.

To get an accurate long-term picture of your blood pressure, you should take the reading at a similar time each day and under similar conditions. To avoid a false high reading, choose a time when you are fairly relaxed. Resting for five minutes beforehand will help.

For best results, observe the following guidelines:

◆ Choose the same time of day to take your blood pressure, whether morning or evening.

◆ Wait half an hour after a cup of coffee or cigarette, as caffeine and nicotine can cause a temporary rise in blood pressure.

◆ Sit comfortably and do a few minutes' calm breathing.

◆ Place the cuff or device on your arm or finger at heart level when you are taking the reading.

DEVICES TO MEASURE BP

There are two main types of device available. The automatic digital type, shown below, displays a reading on a small screen. The aneroid type, which is being used less and less because it is not very accurate, has a dial. For ease of comparison, the measurements produced by these devices are still expressed in millimetres of mercury even though no mercury is used in any of them.

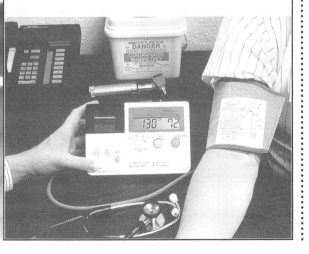

YOU REALLY NEED TO KNOW

◆ There are no set figures at which high BP is diagnosed. It depends on age, lifestyle and existing medical problems.

◆ Some people will need to keep a regular check on their blood pressure.

◆ It's important to follow your doctor's advice on how and when to do it, so you don't become over anxious.

Self monitoring

Getting a diagnosis

If you don't know what your BP is, make an appointment to have it taken.

Anxiety can make your blood pressure rise, so try to relax before having it taken.

Because high blood pressure usually causes no symptoms the only way to find out if yours is normal or not is to have your blood pressure checked regularly. This is increasingly important as you get older, because blood pressure tends to rise with age.

The frequency of checks will vary depending on your health and your doctor's views. (Pregnant women, those taking the oral contraceptive pill and diabetics are special cases; see Chapter 4.) If the doctor thinks you are at a high risk of developing high blood pressure because of your medical history, lifestyle or other factors (see p. 20), he or she may recommend more frequent checks.

HOW OFTEN SHOULD BLOOD PRESSURE BE CHECKED?

AGE	MEN	WOMEN
UP TO 35	Every five years provided you have no other health risks such as obesity.	Every five years provided you have no other health risks, are not pregnant or taking the Pill.
OVER 35	At least every two years or when you visit the doctor's surgery—whichever is the sooner.	Every five years and ideally more often until the menopause. After this every two years or more frequently if using HRT.
DURING PREGNANCY		At every antenatal visit.
IF TAKING THE ORAL CONTRACEPTIVE PILL		Every six months.

FEAR OF DOCTORS

Anxiety can cause your blood pressure to shoot up, so it is important to be as relaxed as possible when you have your blood pressure taken. Some people's blood pressure goes up only when they see the doctor. This is known as "white coat" or "office" hypertension. Doctors do not yet know for certain the import of this. It is known that many people become anxious when visiting the doctor for fear of a worrying diagnosis, and this anxiety alone could cause blood pressure to rise. It is interesting too that some studies have shown that people with white coat hypertension are more likely to have an enlarged heart than those with normal blood pressure, and are more likely to need treatment for high blood pressure.

Ensuring an accurate picture

You won't be diagnosed as having high blood pressure because of the odd high reading. The doctor will usually want to see at least three high readings on three separate occasions over a period of a couple of months before making a firm diagnosis.

If your initial blood pressure reading seems unusually high, the doctor or nurse may take your blood pressure again after you have had a bit of time to relax. If your blood pressure still appears high, you may be asked to return to the surgery for further readings to be taken over the next month or so. Generally blood pressure settles down to the lowest level it is going to reach after around four visits to the surgery. This allows the doctor to decide if you need treatment.

YOU REALLY NEED TO KNOW

◆ Regular blood pressure checks are essential because high blood pressure causes no symptoms.

◆ The doctor won't make a diagnosis until there are three or four separate readings over a period of time.

◆ If you have "white coat hypertension" you may be asked to monitor your BP yourself at home.

Who gets high blood pressure

Try to keep your weight within the ideal range for your height.

Learn some personal strategies for dealing with stress.

If you smoke, make a decision now to quit as soon as you can.

A diet with a lot of processed and junk food will not be healthy because of the high fat, high salt content.

It is not known exactly why some of us are more likely than others to develop high blood pressure but certain factors are known to increase the risk.

Race
Black Africans, African-Caribbean people living in Europe and African-Americans have a higher risk. This may be partly related to the way the body handles salt.

Age
Our blood pressure rises fairly steadily between the ages of 20 and 40. After this it tends to increase more rapidly.

Sex
Women have slightly lower blood pressure than men during their 20s and 30s, but may develop it through hormonal changes, for example in pregnancy (see p. 64) or in using oral contraception. The same can also be true in older women using hormone replacement therapy (HRT) at the menopause.

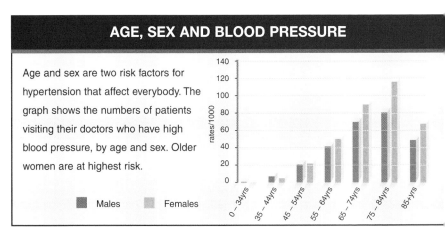

AGE, SEX AND BLOOD PRESSURE

Age and sex are two risk factors for hypertension that affect everybody. The graph shows the numbers of patients visiting their doctors who have high blood pressure, by age and sex. Older women are at highest risk.

■ Males   ■ Females

Family history

f one or both of your parents had high blood pressure you are twice as likely to develop it yourself.

Excess weight

Obesity is a significant risk factor for high blood pressure. Being overweight places strain on the heart.

Diet

A diet high in salt and fat and low in calcium, magnesium and phosphorus has been linked to higher blood pressure. Avoid processed foods and eat more fresh fruit and vegetables.

Stress

The role played by stress in the development of high blood pressure is still uncertain. However, people whose blood pressure soars during stressful situations (the so called "hot reactors") are more likely to go on to develop high blood pressure.

Smoking

Smokers are more likely than non-smokers to develop high blood pressure; nicotine narrows the blood vessels.

Medical conditions

A number of illnesses, many of them hormonal disorders, are linked to hypertension.

Because of their medical condition, people with diabetes already have an even higher risk of suffering stroke, heart and kidney problems. The risk of these possible complications becomes greater when high blood pressure is also a problem.

◆ Some people are more prone than others to developing high blood pressure.

◆ Some of the factors that determine how likely you are to develop high blood pressure are out of your control. Others you can influence.

Who gets high blood pressure?

Effects on the body

SELF HELP

Make sure you have your eyes tested regularly.

Don't ignore symptoms such as dizziness and headaches—see your doctor.

Some doctors call high blood pressure "the silent killer" because it stealthily damages the heart, blood vessels kidneys and other organs with few or no symptoms. In fact about half of all people with high blood pressure are completely unaware of it. Very occasionally, if blood pressure is exceptionally high, people may experience headaches, dizziness and blurred eyesight.

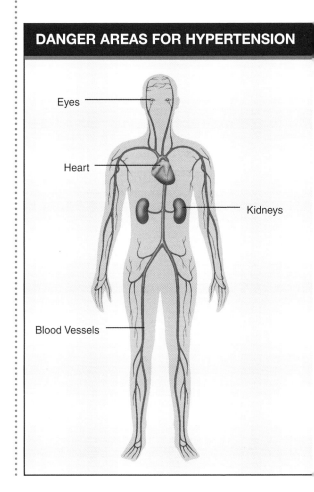

DANGER AREAS FOR HYPERTENSION

Eyes

Heart

Kidneys

Blood Vessels

If your blood pressure is high the doctor will look for signs of organ damage. This involves inspecting the back of your eyes to check for narrowing or thickening of the blood vessels; looking for small haemorrhages inside the eye; listening to your heart to detect any irregularities; checking blood flow in your arteries; and checking the abdomen for signs of kidney enlargement.

EYES

High blood pressure does not seriously damage vision unless it is very high. However, abnormalities in the small blood vessels of the retina can be clearly seen, even in cases of mildly raised blood pressure. It indicates whether blood pressure has been high for some time.

HEART

High blood pressure puts a tremendous strain on the heart. This is partly because less blood is able to reach the heart and also because it forces the heart to work harder to pump blood around the body. Over time, this causes the heart to enlarge and then to weaken and the function deteriorates.

KIDNEYS

High blood pressure damages the tissue and arterioles in the kidneys, causing them to work less efficiently.

BLOOD VESSELS

Untreated high blood pressure causes the blood vessels to narrow and harden and speeds up the development of atherosclerosis, the medical term for furring of the blood vessels, which is linked to heart disease.

YOU REALLY NEED TO KNOW

◆ Blood pressure is known as "the silent killer" because usually it causes no symptoms.

◆ If blood pressure remains high without treatment it can cause a lot of damage.

◆ Blood flow becomes sluggish and the blood becomes thicker and clots more easily.

◆ Prompt treatment reduces the risk of developing serious medical problems.

Effects on the body

Related medical conditions

✓ Report unusual symptoms, such as breathlessness, wheezing, dizziness or loss of memory, to your doctor.

✗ Do not miss regular blood pressure and medical checks after the age of 40.

Because of the damage it causes to the heart and blood vessels, high blood pressure if left untreated can cause a number of medical problems, many of them serious or potentially fatal. Some of these conditions could be avoided simply by having regular blood-pressure checks and appropriate treatment.

Heart failure

The effort of pumping out blood at high pressure puts the heart under stress. Over time, in order to cope with the strain, the heart enlarges. Eventually it begins to fail and the blood supply to the rest of the body decreases. As the condition progresses symptoms include weakness and fatigue. Later, due to the enlargement of the heart, fluid gathers in the lungs and lower limbs causing a cough, breathlessness, swollen feet and ankles.

Kidney failure

Damage to the arterioles obstructs the flow of blood to the kidneys. Eventually the efficiency of kidney function is affected, and they are unable to do the essential job of disposing of waste products, including drugs and alcohol. In the early stages symptoms include nausea, loss of appetite and fatigue.

Poor eyesight

High blood pressure damages the blood vessels in the eyes. This may, in fact, be the first visible clue to the effect high blood pressure is having on other organs. The doctor can see the damage by examining the back of your eye with an instrument called an ophthalmoscope. Extremely high blood pressure can cause hypertensive retinopathy which can lead to blurred vision and blindness.

Stroke

People with high blood pressure are up to seven times more likely to have a stroke. It is estimated that four out of 10 people who die of a stroke could have been saved by having regular blood pressure checks and treatment.

Stroke (sometimes called a brain attack) occurs when the blood supply to the brain is interrupted, usually by a blood clot. Sometimes a stroke occurs when high blood pressure has caused a weak spot in the wall of one of the smaller arteries which bursts. In either case, the affected part of the brain dies, resulting in speech difficulties, loss of vision and paralysis.

Transient ischaemic attack (TIA)

High blood pressure can also cause a transient ischaemic attack (TIA), a mini-stroke, which may cause temporary eyesight disturbances, dizziness and changes in sensation. Although the person returns to normal afterward he or she is more at risk of a true stroke.

Symptoms come on suddenly but are always followed by full recovery. If you suspect that you may have had a TIA, report it to your doctor so that treatment can be prescribed to avert a full stroke.

Dementia

Sometimes a series of "little" strokes, which are not severe but produce sudden physical weakness and double vision, gradually damage the brain tissue. If they continue over a long period, the person may become forgetful and confused. Doctors call this multi-infarct dementia (MID) which may sometimes be confused with Alzheimer's disease. However, in MID drug treatment can slow deterioration.

1

YOU REALLY NEED TO KNOW

◆ Regular blood pressure checks help your doctor monitor your general state of health.

◆ The entire vascular system is at risk if high blood pressure is left untreated.

◆ When the arteries fur up (called atherosclerosis) it can lead to coronary heart disease, heart attacks and peripheral vascular disease.

Related medical conditions

Related medical conditions

Coronary heart disease

If the coronary arteries supplying the heart become hard and inelastic, narrow and furred as a result of high blood pressure, not enough blood gets to the heart. Symptoms can include pain, a feeling of pressure or suffocation in the chest, known as angina, a heart attack or death.

Heart attack

If coronary artery narrows so much that blood is unable to get through to the heart, or if an artery is blocked by a clot becoming lodged in the narrowed arteries, part of the heart is starved of blood and dies. This is a heart attack.

Peripheral vascular disease

When the blood vessels supplying the legs are damaged, insufficient blood reaches the fingers and toes. This in turn can lead to pain in the legs, especially on walking. Peripheral vascular disease may lead to leg ulcers and even gangrene caused by the loss of the blood supply to the feet. This condition is also linked to smoking and diabetes.

HOW THE ARTERIES BECOME FURRED

Arteries have three layers: a smooth inner lining, a muscular layer and a fibrous outer layer. The lining becomes thickened by patches of plaque, reducing the space available for flow of blood.

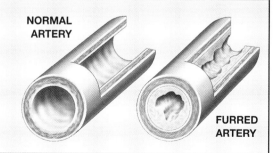

NORMAL ARTERY

FURRED ARTERY

WHAT DOES IT MEAN?

ANGINA

Chest pain or pressure in the chest felt on exertion. It is caused by insufficient blood reaching the heart. Angina may also be felt as pain in the arms or a choking sensation in the neck and throat.

DEMENTIA

Decline in mental ability causing forgetfulness, confusion, mood swings. It can be caused by narrowed or blocked arteries in the brain. Treatment of high blood pressure may slow deterioration.

GANGRENE

Death of tissue, caused by loss of blood supply, for example as a result of acute blockage of the arteries.

ISCHAEMIA

Insufficient supply of blood to an organ or tissue. A transient ischaemic attack (TIA) is when the brain is temporarily starved of blood because of blockage of the arteries supplying the brain. It can cause dizziness and visual disturbances. Ischaemic heart disease (IHD) is caused by blockage of the coronary arteries.

VASCULAR

Meaning of the blood vessels. Peripheral vascular disease is disease in blood vessels far from the heart—in the legs or feet, for example. Like angina, it is caused by an insufficient blood supply to the affected area.

Related medical conditions

Chapter

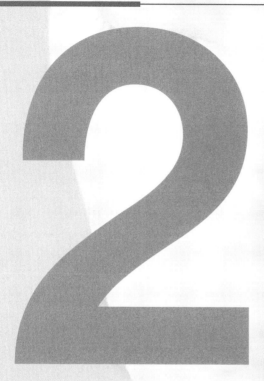

2

TREATMENT & SELF HELP

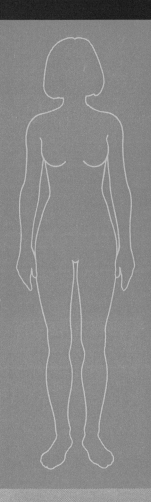

Finding the right treatment

✓ Once you have started treatment, you must return to the doctor for regular blood pressure checks.

✗ It is important that you don't just stop taking your medication. If you are not happy, talk to your doctor about it.

There is a wide range of drugs which your doctor can prescribe to bring your blood pressure down. The aim is to find the particular drug or combination of drugs that will lower your blood pressure to a safe level (ideally to or below 140/85) and prevent problems. The doctor will tailor treatment to you as an individual, so do not be surprised if you find that you are taking completely different drugs to someone else with the same condition.

Why it may take some time

Finding the right drug or combination of drugs may involve a certain amount of trial and error, so be prepared to be patient and to persevere. You will usually be prescribed a low dose of a drug to start with to allow your system to adjust to it and the lower blood pressure. This makes it less likely that you will experience adverse side-effects.

You will be asked to return for regular check-ups to measure the effectiveness of the drug or drugs prescribed. Depending on the results, the doctor may increase your dose or prescribe an additional drug. It is common today to use combination therapy, in which low doses of more than one drug are combined in a single tablet. This is often more effective in controlling blood pressure and produces fewer side-effects than a high dose of a single drug.

Tailoring your medication

Your doctor will tailor your treatment specifically to your needs, selecting the drugs which will deal best with the effects of raised blood pressure on your body. He or she might suggest you keep a diary to note down any side-effects, when they occurred and what they were.

TYPES OF DRUGS

There are different categories of drugs used to bring high blood pressure within a normal range and they work in three different ways.

TYPE 1:
These drugs, known as diuretics, reduce the amount of fluid in the body by increasing urine flow. By reducing body fluid it means that there is less for the heart to pump around the body.

TYPE 2:
Drugs in this category reduce the heart's workload by preventing the stimulating effects of stress, slowing the heartbeat and reducing its force. This makes it easier for the heart to pump blood around the body. Beta blockers are the best known in this category.

TYPE 3:
These act on the widening and narrowing of the blood vessels. The group includes ACE inhibitors, which block the formation of the hormone angiotensin that causes the blood vessels to narrow; angiotensin II inhibitors which block the effect of angiotensin; calcium channel blockers, which relax the blood vessels; and alpha blockers which also relax the blood vessels.

Drug treatment for hypertension is not short term. It may be necessary for some years or for the rest of your life, but controlling the condition is likely to give you more years of good health than bad.

2

YOU REALLY NEED TO KNOW

◆ Finding the correct treatment may take some time and you may have to be patient.

◆ Combination therapy—taking two types of drugs in a single tablet—is often extremely successful and produces fewer side-effects.

◆ Different kinds of blood-pressure lowering drugs work on the body in different ways.

Finding the right treatment

Medication charts

The charts on the following pages show the various types of different drugs that may be prescribed and explain how they work and what side-effects they may have.

TYPE 1 AND TYPE 2 DRUGS

DRUG	HOW THEY WORK
DIURETICS ("WATER TABLETS")	Work on kidneys to increase output of urine, reduce volume of circulating blood. (Unlikely to be the main medium of action in the long term.)
BETA BLOCKERS	Block the action of stress hormones produced by the body which make the heart beat faster, thus slowing the heart rate and reducing the work that the heart has to do. This reduces the amount of oxygen the heart needs and improves its ability to cope with physical exertion.

POSSIBLE SIDE-EFFECTS	GENERIC NAMES
Loss of appetite	bendrofluazide
Stomach upsets	chlorthalidone
Dehydration	indapamide
Impotence	metolazone
Increased cholesterol level	
Allergic reactions	
Increased uric acid (leading to risk of gout)	
Raised blood sugar	
Light headedness	oxprenolol
Pins and needles	propranolol
Cold fingers and toes	atenolol
Stomach upsets	bisoprolol
Depression	nadolol
Nightmares	indalol
Wheezing	imolol
Drowsiness	
Lethargy	
Weakness	
Fatigue	
Visual disturbances	

YOU REALLY NEED TO KNOW

◆ Diuretics and beta blockers used to be the first line treatment for high blood pressure, but are less frequently prescribed today.

◆ Different people respond to drugs in different ways.

◆ Beta blockers should never be stopped abruptly. The dose should be gradually reduced over several weeks.

Medication charts

Medication charts

The drugs on this medication chart all act by affecting the mechanism by which the arteries widen and narrow. Widening the arteries allows more blood through so is an effective way of lowering blood pressure.

TYPE 3 DRUGS

DRUG	HOW THEY WORK
ACE INHIBITORS (ANGIOTENSIN-CONVERTING ENZYME INHIBITORS)	Block formation of the hormone angiotensin II, which causes the blood vessels to narrow. The action of this drug improves blood flow and therefore decreases the amount of work the heart has to do. More salt and water are lost in urine as well.
CALCIUM CHANNEL BLOCKERS (CALCIUM ANTAGONISTS)	Reduces the amount of calcium in muscles which form the walls of the arteries, relaxing them and causing arteries to widen. This leads to a drop in blood pressure. It also reduces the workload of the heart and cuts down its oxygen needs.

POSSIBLE SIDE-EFFECTS	GENERIC NAMES
Coughing	gaptopril
Dizziness on sitting or standing up (postural hypotension)	enalapril
	lisinopril
	ramipril
General dizziness	
Rash	
Allergic reactions	
Loss of taste	
Flushing	amlodipine
Headache	diltiazem
Swollen ankles	nifedipine
Dizziness	verapamil
Other rare side-effects:	
Fatigue	
Nausea	
Palpitations	
Drowsiness	
Insomnia	
Stomach upsets	
Rashes	
Ringing in the ears	

2

YOU REALLY NEED TO KNOW

◆ ACE inhibitors and calcium channel blockers taken in combination seem to have a protective effect on organs such as the kidneys.

◆ Calcium channel blockers appear to be especially effective in lowering blood pressure for African, African-Caribbean and older people.

Medication charts

Medication charts

The drugs on this medication chart all work by blocking the action of different hormones involved in the widening and narrowing of the arteries.

TYPE 2 AND TYPE 3 DRUGS

TYPE OF DRUG	HOW THEY WORK
ANGIOTENSIN II ANTAGONISTS	Block the hormone angiotensin II, which narrows the blood vessels, in the kidneys, adrenal glands, heart, brain and sympathetic nervous system.
ALPHA BLOCKERS	Block effects of stress hormones in the arteries, causing the arteries to widen and reducing resistance to the flow of blood.
ALPHA-BETA BLOCKERS	Block effects of stress hormones. Widen arteries and reduce resistance to flow of blood. Also slow heartbeat so less blood is pumped through system.

POSSIBLE SIDE-EFFECTS	GENERIC NAMES
Dizziness	irbesartan
	losartan
Dizziness on standing (postural hypotension)	doxazosin
	prazosin
Vertigo	terazosin
Headache	
Lack of energy	
Palpitations	
Passing urine more often	
Fluid retention and swelling (oedema)	
As alpha blockers (above) and beta blockers (pp. 34–35)	labetalol
	carvedilol

YOU REALLY NEED TO KNOW

◆ Alpha blockers are especially useful for people with diabetes, and kidney damage.

◆ Because alpha blockers help relax the bladder, they may help men with prostate problems, but can cause urinary incontinence in women.

Taking your medication

Make sure you know what your medication is for and how you should take it.

Try to get into a routine that makes it easy to remember when to take your drugs.

Even if you feel well do not stop taking your medication. Make an appointment to see your doctor or nurse to discuss it.

For drug treatment of high blood pressure to be effective, it is important that you understand your doctor's instructions clearly and follow them carefully.

What your doctor should tell you

Before leaving the doctor's surgery, make sure you understand exactly what the drug has been prescribed for and what side effects you can expect. Ask your

YOUR MEDICATION ROUTINE

If you find it difficult to keep track of what you have taken and when, and especially if you have to take several different types of drugs, you may find it useful to get a special drugs dispenser. These are designed to help you organize your drugs and remember when to take them. Always check the label for the expiry date of your drugs, and discard any that you have not used by this date.

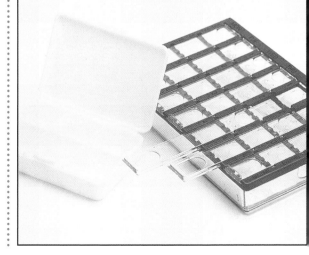

QUESTIONS TO ASK THE DOCTOR

◆ When should I take the drug?

◆ What can I eat or drink when I take the drug?

◆ Should I take the drug with a meal?

◆ Are there any other drugs I cannot take with this drug?

◆ What should I do if I run out of the drug?

◆ What should I do if I forget to take a dose?

YOU REALLY NEED TO KNOW

◆ You may need frequent check-ups until your doctor is satisfied that your drug regime is working.

◆ You may find it helpful to use a special medication dispenser to keep track of when to take your drugs.

◆ Ask the doctor or pharmacist if there are any special instructions connected to taking your drugs.

doctor how many times a day you need to take the drug, and when and how it should be taken. Most tablets or capsules are best taken with fluid or they might lodge in your gullet, which can delay absorption.

When you pick up the prescription, ask the pharmacist if there are any special instructions, though these will be written on the packet or in the accompanying leaflet.

Follow-up

Your doctor should tell you how often you will have to return to the surgery for check-ups. You are likely to have to go for more frequent check-ups at first until he or she is satisfied that the right prescription for you has been found. Once the doctor is satisfied that the medication is working with as few side-effects as possible the number of visits you have to make to the surgery will decrease.

If you are in any doubt about any drug you have been prescribed, discuss your concerns with your doctor or pharmacist.

Dealing with side-effects

✓ Always report any side-effects you experience to the doctor.

✓ Keep a note of what happened, when it occurred and how severe it was.

✗ Don't forget to ask if the medication will clash with drugs you may be taking for another condition.

All drugs have side-effects as well as benefits. For example if you are prescribed a diuretic you will usually find you need to pass urine more often, especially when you first start taking the drug.

It is a good idea to know what side-effects are likely so that if you do develop any of them you can report them to your doctor. The good news is that, with new developments in drugs, the likelihood of experiencing side-effects is becoming less. The side-effects listed on the charts on pages 32–37 are those which are commonly linked to the various medications outlined. When listed in this way, they can appear off-putting, but you should bear in mind that many side-effects are mild and wear off once your body has got used to the drug.

Weigh up the benefits

If you think you are experiencing a side-effect it is vitally important that you do not suddenly stop taking the drug that you believe may be the cause. Instead, make an appointment to see your doctor as soon as possible so you can discuss it. The doctor will try to weigh up the benefits of the drug against the disadvantage of any side-effects and may change the dosage or prescribe a different drug. Try to be patient. It may take a while to find the precise dosage or drug that is best for you.

Finding ways to cope

Some side-effects are more of a nuisance than serious, and you may be able to get round them with a few self-help measures. If lack of energy is a problem, for example, you could try pacing yourself, paying attention to your eating habits and adding in some daily exercise to help improve your energy levels.

Other side-effects ease off after a short period so you may need simply to bear it until they do. Your doctor can advise you on how long this should take. If the side-effect does not disappear within a reasonable period, he or she will usually be able to prescribe another drug.

If this isn't possible you may have to accept that putting up with a few minor side-effects is part of getting your health right. It can be hard to see why you need to continue taking a drug that is causing you to feel ill and it will help to keep in mind the greater health benefits of controlling your blood pressure.

Work as a team

It is important to establish a trusting relationship with your doctor and work with him or her discover your ideal medication regime. You should always feel free to ask questions and it will help if you make your appointments for less busy times so there is time for you to talk.

◆ It may take some time for your body to get used to the drug or drugs prescribed.

◆ Some side-effects are merely a nuisance, others are more troublesome.

◆ When you report any side-effects you experience to the doctor, it may not always be possible to change your prescription.

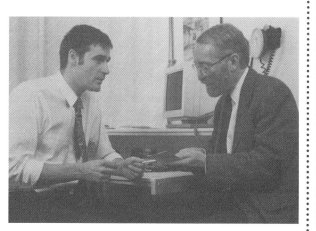

Regular sessions with your doctor are part of being treated for high blood pressure. Assessing how the drugs are working and your response to them will involve both of you as a team.

Dealing with side-effects

Treatment with aspirin

Aspirin is often prescribed for people with controlled high blood pressure. It is not used for its pain relieving qualities, but helps reduce the risk of heart attacks and other cardiovascular complications.

Strokes and heart attacks

Most people who have had a stroke, mini-strokes (TIAs) or heart attack will be prescribed a mini-dose of aspirin to help protect against a repeat of the problem. The mini-dose is one 75 mg tablet daily, about a quarter of a standard aspirin tablet.

Aspirin does not act directly on the blood pressure. Instead it helps to lower the risk of blood clots forming by reducing the stickiness of platelets, special blood cells that are involved in the clotting process. If a clot forms in the arteries leading to the brain this can cause a stroke or TIA, while a clot in the coronary arteries can cause a heart attack.

HOT TREATMENT

Aspirin is derived from willow bark, and its pain relieving and anti-inflammatory effects have been recognized for a century. However, it is only relatively recently that its anti-clotting properties have been put to use in the treatment of heart disease. An international study, known as the Hypertension Optimal Treatment (HOT) trial found that combining a small dose of aspirin with blood-pressure-lowering drugs in people with high blood pressure reduced the risk of heart attacks by as much as 36 percent.

PLATELETS AND BLOOD VESSELS

Platelets are the smallest blood cells and they play an important role in clotting. Normally, clotting is a useful function–if you suffer a wound of the skin, for example, clotting stops you from bleeding to death and seals the area to prevent infection entering.

Problems arise, however, inside the body when platelets come into contact with damaged areas on the blood vessel walls (which may have been caused by prolonged and untreated high BP). The blood flow becomes more turbulent, the clotting process is triggered leading to unwanted blood clots, or thrombi, which are involved in thrombosis, the medical word for abnormal clot formation. If a thrombus forms in a blood vessel supplying the heart or the brain, it can cause a heart attack or stroke.

Preventative action

Aspirin is known medically as an anti-platelet drug. By working chemically on the platelets, a type of red blood cell involved in the process of clotting, aspirin makes blood clots more slippery so they do not lodge in the blood vessels and cause a stroke or heart attack.

Aspirin is sometimes prescribed for people who have angina, pain caused by heart disease. Other anti-platelet drugs may be prescribed instead of or as well as aspirin. You should never however take aspirin in this way unless under medical supervision.

After a stroke or heart attack, the risk of another occurring is greatest in the next few months, so the sooner preventative treatment is begun the better.

YOU REALLY NEED TO KNOW

◆ Aspirin is prescribed as routine for people who have had a stroke or a heart attack and often for someone who has had a mini-stroke (TIA).

◆ Aspirin does not treat high blood pressure directly.

◆ People with diabetes have to be careful as large amounts of aspirin can alter blood glucose levels. However, a dose given for high blood pressure is always very small.

Treatment with aspirin

Will I always need medication?

Taking blood-pressure lowering medication can lower the risk of stroke by 35–40%.

Taking blood-pressure lowering medication can reduce the likelihood of developing heart disease by 20–25%.

Research shows that taking blood-pressure-lowering medication can dramatically cut your risk of having a stroke and developing heart disease, so it really is well worth carrying on taking it.

If you are prescribed drugs to control your blood pressure, you will probably have to take them for the rest of your life. It can be difficult to accept this, especially if you feel perfectly well or if you are experiencing troublesome side-effects.

In a minority of cases it may be possible to gradually stop medication. But if you do it against your doctor's advice your risk of developing serious complications such as heart attack or stroke will rise dramatically. Your blood pressure may become harder to control and you could end up taking even more drugs.

What if I improve my lifestyle?

Making diet and lifestyle changes (see Chapter Three) is one of the most important things you can do to help lower your blood pressure. Research has proved that a combination of lifestyle measures and drug treatment lowers blood pressure in over eight out of 10 sufferers and dramatically reduces the risk of complications.

However, lifestyle changes alone will be enough in only a very few cases. If your high blood pressure was mild and you only needed minimal medication, you may be able to control your blood pressure sufficiently in this way. Nevertheless, about half of all people who stop taking blood-pressure-lowering drugs have to start taking them again at a later date.

If your doctor does consider your blood pressure to be sufficiently well controlled for you to be able to stop taking medication you will still need regular check-ups.

ROUTINE CHECKS

Once you are settled on your medication and your blood pressure is under control, you will have to return to the doctor's surgery regularly to have your blood pressure checked. These routine checks are often performed by the nurse rather than the doctor.

◆ You will usually need to have your blood pressure checked about four times a year once it has stabilized.

◆ It is vital that you attend your check-ups to make sure that your blood pressure remains under control.

◆ The doctor may recommend other checks from time to time, perhaps at the hospital, to make sure that your heart, blood vessels and kidneys are healthy.

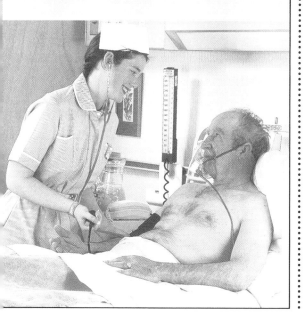

**YOU REALLY
NEED TO KNOW**

◆ Only occasionally can lifestyle measures lower blood pressure sufficiently for you to stop taking medication.

◆ If you stop taking medication without your doctor's advice your blood pressure may rise dangerously and become harder to control.

Will I always need medication?

Chapter

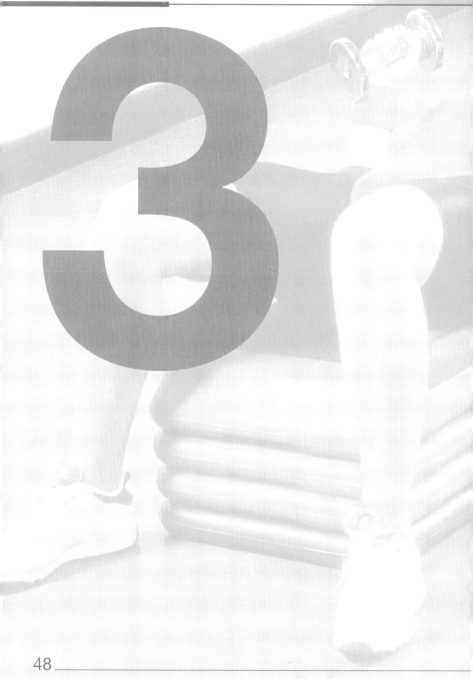

DAY TO DAY
LIFESTYLE

Weight control

SELF HELP

Diet with a friend or join a slimming club to help increase your motivation.

Avoid crash diets and miracle solutions. Instead aim to lose weight gradually—it is more likely to stay off that way.

Excess weight increases the work your heart has to do in pumping blood around your body. If you are overweight you are also more likely to have high cholesterol and to develop diabetes—both of which increase your risk of having heart disease or a stroke. These risks are even greater in women than in men. Weight control is believed by many experts to be an important factor in reducing the risk of high blood pressure.

Losing weight will help to lower your blood pressure and reduce your risk of having a stroke, heart attack or other serious illnesses. Research has found that for every kilogram of weight you lose your blood pressure will fall by one millimetre of mercury. If your blood pressure is only slightly raised, shedding excess pounds may return it to normal without the need for medication.

WHY A HEALTHY DIET IS THE BEST WEIGHT-LOSS DIET

The best way to lose weight is gradually. On a low-calorie diet your body, thinking it is starved of food, raids the muscles for the fuel stored there (this is the first weight you lose) and this saps your energy. Your metabolism slows down.
On a healthy diet, a steady reduction in weight occurs as stored fat is burnt up, your muscle increases and you also have a lot more energy.

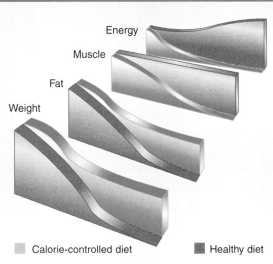

Energy
Muscle
Fat
Weight

Calorie-controlled diet   Healthy diet

EFFECTIVE WEIGHT LOSS

◆ Aim to lose weight slowly—half to one kilogram a week.

◆ The best way to lose weight is to cut down on fatty and sugary foods and eat more fresh fruit and vegetables.

◆ Weight-loss diets work better if combined with exercise.

How to lose weight

The food you eat provides your body with energy. Ideally, you should not take in any more than your body can use. If you do consume more, you will put on weight because the body turns excess to fat which it stores.

To lose weight you need to put into your mouth fewer calories than you burn up (a calorie is simply a unit of energy). The best way to lose weight is to eat less and burn up more calories through increasing the amount of physical activity you do.

If your doctor feels you need to lose weight, you may be given a diet sheet to follow. If you have more than a few pounds to lose, you may be referred to a dietitian who can advise you on a sensible, healthy eating plan.

Get support

Some people find it hard to persevere with a long-term weight-loss programme. If you are one of them it may help to join a slimming club, where you will get advice on how to keep up your weight-loss plans and support from other people with a common goal. If you are struggling to maintain a healthy eating regime, try to keep in mind how much better you will feel once you have lost weight.

YOU REALLY NEED TO KNOW

◆ Excess weight forces your heart to work harder and increases your risk of heart disease, stroke and diabetes.

◆ Every kilo of weight you lose has a direct effect on lowering your blood pressure.

◆ The best way to lose weight is through a combination of diet and exercise.

Weight control

What to eat and drink

✓ Aim to eat at least five servings of fruit and vegetables a day.

✗ Avoid eating processed foods and do not add salt to your food at the table. Try using herbs, spices and lemon to season foods instead.

✗ Sea salt, rock salt and natural salt are as bad for raised blood pressure as ordinary table or cooking salt.

What you eat and drink has a major effect on your blood pressure. In particular, reducing the amount of salt (sodium chloride) and fatty foods and increasing the amount of fruit and vegetables you eat can help lower your blood pressure and prevent high blood pressure from developing.

Bypass the salt

An excess of salt in the diet can increase blood pressure. Processed foods such as burgers, sausages, salted snacks, canned vegetables and meats, stock cubes, sauces and ready-made meals contain a lot of salt, so cut down on these and eat more fresh fruit, vegetables, meat and fish instead. When buying prepared foods, check the labels and choose those labelled "low sodium" or "unsalted". Avoid adding salt to your food when you cook and at the table. Low salt, which is a third sodium chloride and two thirds potassium chloride, is available as a healthier alternative.

If you persevere with a low salt diet, you will gradually find that you lose your taste for it after a month or so. If you really can't do without it, however, there are salt substitutes available. These should be used with care if you are taking diuretics or your kidneys are not working well. Ask your doctor to advise you.

Cut down on fat

Doctors and scientists do not yet know whether eating a high-fat diet raises blood pressure. However, a high fat intake (especially the saturated fat found in animal products) can raise blood cholesterol levels, which in turn increases your risk of heart disease. In particular, avoid fatty meat and full-fat dairy products such as pork pies, sausages, burgers and cheese.

WHAT DOES IT MEAN?

ANTIOXIDANTS

Chemicals found in fruit and vegetables that help to protect the body's cells against damage from free radicals.

CHOLESTEROL

A natural waxy substance made by the liver and essential for cells. In some people an excess builds up in the blood and contributes to the furring of the arteries linked to heart disease and stroke.

FREE RADICALS

Rogue molecules produced in the body by normal processes such as breathing and digestion. Their chemical action on cells causes damage that is thought to be an important factor in heart disease and stroke.

SATURATED FAT

The type of fat found in fatty meats, poultry (especially the skin), milk, butter, cream, cheese and many bought baked goods (pastry, biscuits). It solidifies at room temperature.

SODIUM CHLORIDE

The chemical name for salt.

More fruit and vegetables

Fresh fruit and vegetables contain chemicals called antioxidants which help mop up other chemicals called free radicals which cause damage to blood vessels. Fruit and vegetables also contain the mineral potassium, which may also lower blood pressure. Aim to eat at least five servings of fruit and vegetables every day.

YOU REALLY NEED TO KNOW

◆ Read the list of ingredients on bought foods. Avoid any where salt, sugar or fat are high on the list.

◆ Eating fewer fatty foods helps reduce cholesterol levels and lowers the risk of heart disease.

◆ Eating a wide variety of fruit and vegetables every day can help protect against high blood pressure.

What to eat and drink

53

Moderate drinking

Try to drink with food or intersperse drinks with water.

Ask your doctor about drinking if you have had a stroke or heart attack.

Keep to sensible drinking levels and aim to have one or two alcohol-free days every week.

Be aware of the alcohol content of what you are drinking. Some canned and bottled beers are twice as strong as ordinary ones.

Don't binge. You should never drink all your weekly alcohol units at once. Spread them out over several days.

While a small amount of alcohol is believed by some experts to help protect against heart disease, regularly drinking too much can raise your blood pressure and increase your chance of having a stroke. Drinking a lot all at once (bingeing) is especially harmful. In fact, it can increase your risk of having a stroke or cerebral haemorrhage fivefold. This is because it can cause blood pressure to rise steeply, which in turn increases the risk of a blood vessel bursting and bleeding into your brain.

It is also worth bearing in mind, if you are trying to lose weight, that alcoholic drinks can be measured in calories—which may be another good reason to keep your consumption moderate.

KNOW YOUR ALCOHOL UNITS

One unit of alcohol is equivalent to one small drink. That is about a small glass (125 ml) of wine, a single pub measure of spirits or half a pint (300 ml) of weak beer or lager. With stronger beers or wines, a unit may be significantly more. For example, a small glass of fortified wine contains one and a half units of alcohol.

Women are advised to keep alcohol intake to two to three units of drink a day—no more than 14 a week. Men should keep alcohol intake to no more than four units a day—no more than 21 a week.

Learn to keep track of what you are drinking so that you know when you have had your number of units.

Beware, especially in restaurants—it is all too easy to just keep topping up your glass and to go over your limit without really being aware of it.

Sensible drinking

Sticking to sensible drinking levels and avoiding binges can help to reduce your blood pressure and lower your risk of having a heart attack or stroke. Follow the recommendations for men and women (below), and spread your drinking through the week rather than drinking your weekly allowance in one or two sessions. Aim to have one or two alcohol-free days every week.

Try to drink slowly, sipping your drink and fully appreciating the flavour, rather than just knocking it back. Take the edge off your thirst with a soft drink first so that you do not gulp down your drink. Also try to intersperse alcohol with soft drinks.

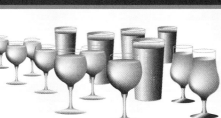

Maximum weekly consumption for women = 14 units

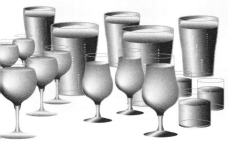

Maximum weekly consumption for men = 21 units

Moderate drinking

Enjoying exercise

✓ Aim to do something active most days— choose a form of exercise or activity that you enjoy.

✓ Start slowly and build up gradually so you won't become bored.

✗ Don't overdo it. Avoid very competitive or vigorous forms of sport such as squash or weight training.

✗ Don't go for the "burn". Exercise does not have to hurt to do you good, and you risk injury, which will disrupt your exercise programme.

Lack of physical activity can increase your blood pressure, and lead to weight gain. Taking regular exercise can lower your blood pressure and will also help you to control your weight. It will make you look and feel better, and has even been found to help relieve depression.

How much exercise?

If you have not exercised recently and have been diagnosed with high blood pressure (especially if you are taking medication) or have had a stroke or heart attack, you should check with your doctor before embarking on an exercise programme. You could seek the help of a

HOW EXERCISE HELPS

Regular aerobic exercise, the kind which uses oxygen and makes you feel out of breath, helps strengthen your heart and improves its ability to pump blood, so reducing its overall workload. Aerobic exercise also helps to burn fat.

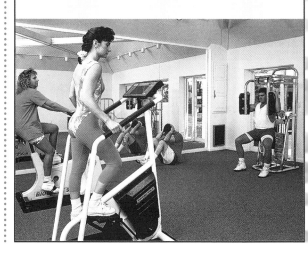

local gym to help you achieve 30 minutes of moderate physical activity on at least five days a week. If this seems daunting, or if you are short of time, it is not necessary to do the 30 minutes at once—you could break it into three 10-minute sessions, for example.

What kind of exercise?

Any physical activity will do from a brisk walk to gardening or housework, as long as you get warm and slightly out of breath. If you can't manage that at first, do whatever you can and build up gradually.

One way to fulfil your exercise quota could be simply to incorporate more activity into your daily life—by walking rather than taking a bus, for example, or climbing the stairs rather than taking an escalator or lift. This kind of approach is particularly useful for people who feel they don't have time to exercise. Practically the only thing to avoid if you have high blood pressure is competitive or vigorous exercise such as marathon running, squash, press-ups or weight training.

Keeping it up

It is important to keep up your exercise programme, even if your blood pressure goes down. If you stop, your blood pressure may return to its previous level. If you find it hard to stay motivated, you may find it helps to exercise with a friend. Exercise is more enjoyable if you have company, and you are less likely to be tempted to skip, say, a swimming session if you've made an arrangement to meet your friend at the pool. You could also vary your activities to add interest—for example, you could go for a walk three days a week and swim, cycle, play badminton or tennis or do some gardening on the others.

YOU REALLY NEED TO KNOW

◆ Regular exercise can help lower your blood pressure, reduce weight and make you look and feel better.

◆ Everyday activities such as walking can form part of an exercise programme.

◆ It is important to maintain your exercise programme or you will lose the benefits.

Quitting smoking

Start now. The benefits of giving up smoking are immediate and they increase with time.

Don't feel that all is lost if you slip up sometimes. Just congratulate yourself that you have done well so far and carry on trying.

Smoking increases the risk of heart attack, stroke and other arterial disease. If you smoke you are at least twice as likely to suffer a stroke as someone who does not smoke, and five times more likely to develop heart disease. In the UK, it is estimated that 24 percent of deaths from coronary heart disease in men and 11 percent in women are due to smoking.

The effects on your body

Every puff you take on a cigarette acts on the blood vessels and causes them to constrict. Over time, smoking causes furring and narrowing of the arteries and makes your blood more likely to clot—both of which increase your risk of heart disease and stroke. What is more, smoking multiplies the dangers of other risk factors such as diabetes and high blood cholesterol levels, especially in women.

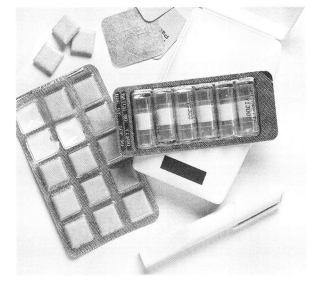

There are plenty of aids to help you quit smoking, including patches, chewing gums and sprays. These work by allowing you gradually to lose your nicotine dependence.

FIVE STEPS TO SUCCESS

◆ Keep in mind the benefits of giving up smoking.

◆ Take it one step at a time.

◆ Ask your doctor about nicotine patches and other aids.

◆ Enlist the support of your family and friends on your side and ask your doctor about help that is available locally.

◆ Avoid situations where you routinely have a cigarette. For example, if you usually have one with a mid-morning coffee, change your routine to break the habit.

The good news is that if you quit, no matter how long you have been a smoker, your risks go down. Giving up smoking will halve your risk of stroke.

Ways to give up

Quitting smoking is not always easy but there are lots of things you can do to help yourself. Giving up with a friend or relative can help keep up your motivation and many surgeries now run special groups for people wanting to stop smoking. Nicotine chewing gums, sprays and patches can also help quell the craving for a cigarette. Ask your doctor about them.

Think about your daily routine, pinpointing the times when you are most likely to light up. Consider what changes you could make. Starting an exercise routine can have a calming effect and improve your feel-good factor. Stress reduction techniques may also help you to deal with the tension caused by giving up.

YOU REALLY NEED TO KNOW

◆ Smoking has a direct effect on the walls of blood vessels and therefore on blood pressure.

◆ In women it multiplies the dangers of diabetes and high cholesterol levels.

◆ Over time smoking contributes to furring and narrowing of the arteries and makes your blood more likely to clot.

◆ Giving up will bring immediate and long-term benefits.

Quitting smoking

Managing stress

Put yourself first. Schedule a little time every day to relax.

Learn some problem-solving skills so that you feel more in control of stressful situations.

Don't waste time worrying about things that you can't change.

Feeling anxious or tense pushes up your blood pressure in the short term because stress causes the release of hormones that narrow your blood vessels and force your heart to beat harder. Even so, doctors are still not sure whether long-term stress is harmful to the blood vessels.

A sense of control

Researchers have discovered that the amount of control people feel they have over their lives can affect physical health. Those who feel more out of control tend to have higher blood pressure and are more likely to experience heart attacks. The results seem to imply that learning to approach life's inevitable ups-and-downs in a practical, constructive way may lower your blood pressure.

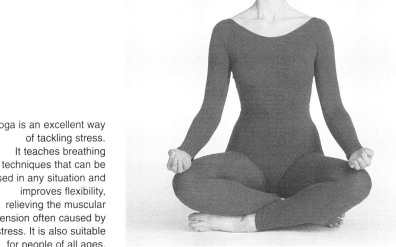

Yoga is an excellent way of tackling stress. It teaches breathing techniques that can be used in any situation and improves flexibility, relieving the muscular tension often caused by stress. It is also suitable for people of all ages.

DEALING WITH YOUR WORRIES

If you are a habitual worrier, learning effective ways to deal with problems can help you feel more in control.

◆ Define the problem.

◆ Make a list of possible solutions.

◆ Select the solutions that are most practical.

◆ Enlist any support you need.

◆ Put your plan into action.

◆ Think positively.

Make time to relax

A balance between work, rest and play is important. Try to build time for relaxation into your daily life. Many busy people feel they don't have time for it, but you will work more productively and efficiently if you are relaxed. Stopping to relax can be a better investment than spending half an hour tackling a problem when you are too tired and stressed to think straight.

Resting your mind

Relaxation does not necessarily mean doing nothing. For example, someone watching television may actually be thinking through their problems. Active pursuits such as gardening or dancing can be restful because they take your mind off your problems and help to disperse stress hormones. Studies have also shown that meditation can lower blood pressure while you are doing it.

YOU REALLY NEED TO KNOW

◆ Stress forces the heart to beat harder and pushes up blood pressure in the short term.

◆ People who feel they have little control over their lives often have high blood pressure.

◆ It is important to make time for regular relaxation and pursuits that you enjoy.

◆ Physical activity can be relaxing and can reduce stress levels.

Managing stress

Chapter

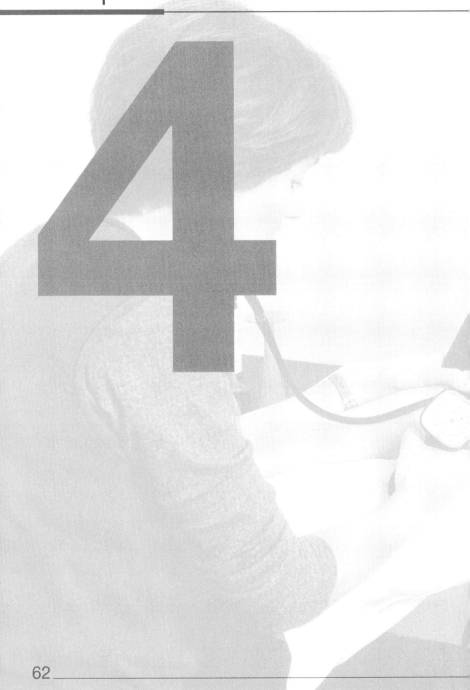

SPECIAL CASES

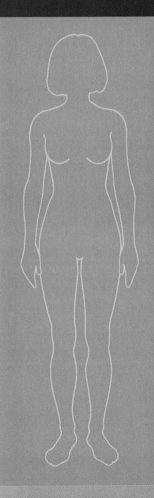

Pregnancy

It helps to go to bed earlier so that you get at least eight hours sleep a night.

Try not to worry. Mildly raised blood pressure will not usually harm your baby.

Don't miss your check-ups and antenatal visits.

Pregnancy causes enormous changes in the amount of blood flowing around the body and in blood pressure. This is partly because the heart beats faster and partly because the hormones of pregnancy cause the blood vessels to relax.

During the first 20 weeks of pregnancy, blood pressure remains the same or lower than before the pregnancy. After this it drops as the blood vessels in the body dilate and the placenta pumps blood to the baby. During the first few months fainting and dizziness can sometimes be a problem due to low blood pressure.

Why your BP is monitored

Blood pressure measurement is one of the routine tests carried out at every antenatal check-up. This is because a raised blood pressure during pregnancy can sometimes be a sign of a serious disease called pre-eclampsia (see p. 66). Treatment of high blood pressure in pregnancy depends on when it begins. If it occurs after 28 weeks, it is likely to be a sign of pre-eclampsia and immediate action must be taken.

Possible treatment

If you have high blood pressure in early pregnancy it may be that your blood pressure was high before you became pregnant but you were not aware of it.

If your blood pressure is only mildly raised, the doctor may advise lifestyle measures and rest to help improve the blood supply to the baby. You will have frequent checks and the doctor will try to decide whether you need drug treatment.

If your blood pressure is severely raised you will usually need to be admitted to hospital for tests to check

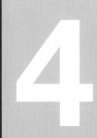

4

WHAT DOES IT MEAN?

PLACENTA

An organ that forms in the uterus during pregnancy and to which the growing foetus is attached by the umbilical cord. The placenta is rich in blood vessels through which the foetus receives its blood supply from the mother.

ANTENATAL VISIT

Routine medical check-up during pregnancy to monitor the health of mother and baby. These may take place once a month early in the pregnancy, increasing to once a week towards the end.

for problems such as kidney disease or diabetes. Careful checks will be made to make sure the problem is not affecting your kidneys and tests will be performed to make sure that your baby is growing properly. Medication to lower blood pressure will be prescribed if necessary, though some drugs are unsuitable.

Self help during pregnancy

If you are found to have raised blood pressure ask your doctor what it is safe for you to do. In general you should try to get as much rest as possible, in the day as well as at night, and avoid any prolonged or vigorous exercise. Eat a sensible diet with plenty of fresh fruit and vegetables, whole grains, lean meat and fish.

Lying on one side when in bed can help improve blood supply to your baby by reducing pressure on the large arteries that lead to the uterus.

YOU REALLY NEED TO KNOW

◆ A pregnant woman has 2litres (3 pints) more blood flowing around her body.

◆ Low blood pressure can be a problem in early pregnancy, causing fainting.

◆ Blood pressure should be measured at every antenatal visit during pregnancy.

◆ If blood pressure is severely raised, hospital admission is usually needed to check for problems such as kidney disease or diabetes.

Pregnancy

Pre-eclampsia

✓ Pre-eclampsia affects 25% of women during their first pregnancy.

✓ Women over 30 are more at risk of developing pre-eclampsia.

✓ Pre-eclampsia usually disappears completely within a few weeks of birth.

About one in four women expecting their first baby develops a condition called pre-eclampsia, which is characterized by high blood pressure. It can also occur in subsequent pregnancies, though this is less common. The condition disappears when the baby is born. The doctor may advise bed rest and possibly drug treatment as well.

What are the symptoms?

A steep rise in blood pressure to 140/90 or more after 28 weeks of pregnancy together with swollen ankles, hands or feet, a sudden weight gain and protein in the urine are signs of pre-eclampsia. It is not known exactly what causes this condition, but it is thought to be due to an abnormality of the placenta. If left untreated, pre-eclampsia can develop into eclampsia, a dangerous condition that can cause convulsions and threaten the lives of both mother and baby.

If you have pre-eclampsia you will be admitted to hospital so that you and your baby can be monitored.

WHO GETS PRE-ECLAMPSIA?

The condition is more common:

◆ In a first pregnancy

◆ If your mother had it

◆ If you are expecting twins

◆ If you have diabetes

◆ If you are overweight.

DANGER SIGNS

Contact your doctor immediately if you are in the late stages of pregnancy and experience any of the following signs which can indicate increased blood pressure:

◆ A sudden severe headache

◆ Visual disturbance

◆ Abdominal pain.

The only real cure is delivery of the baby. If your blood pressure continues to rise or the baby's growth is being affected, the doctor may decide to deliver your baby early. You will usually be offered epidural anaesthesia during labour as this lowers the blood pressure.

Follow-up

In most women their blood pressure comes down after the baby's birth and they experience no further problems. (Pre-eclampsia is less common in second and subsequent pregnancies.) Sometimes, however, blood pressure stays raised and treatment and further tests may be needed.

There is also evidence that some women who have had pre-eclampsia have a higher risk of developing high blood pressure in later life. For this reason it is a good idea to ask your doctor to check your blood pressure every year if you suffered from pre-eclampsia during pregnancy. You should know what the risks of developing it again are before trying for another baby.

YOU REALLY NEED TO KNOW

◆ A sudden rise in blood pressure, swelling and protein in the urine are signs of pre-eclampsia.

◆ Pre-eclampsia is a potentially dangerous condition that affects only pregnant women.

◆ If you have had pre-eclampsia you may be prone to high blood pressure in later life.

Pre-eclampsia

The pill and HRT

Both oral contraceptives, popularly called the pill, and hormone replacement therapy (HRT) can affect blood pressure. Each has differing amounts of the female sex hormone oestrogen which is thought to be the cause.

Taking contraception

The combined contraceptive pill, which contains oestrogen and progestogen, can cause a small rise in blood pressure which is usually not of any importance. A few women, however (around 5 percent), experience a rise in diastolic blood pressure to over 90 mm Hg; very occasionally there may be a more severe rise. The problem is more likely to occur in women who are over 35, are overweight, smoke or have a previous history of high blood pressure. Your doctor may recommend low-oestrogen or progestogen-only pills, which are less likely to cause problems.

You may be able to take the pill even if you have high blood pressure, provided you have regular blood pressure checks. Ask your doctor for advice.

At the menopause

HRT is prescribed to help with symptoms of the menopause caused by reduced oestrogen levels, such as hot flushes, vaginal dryness, mood swings and reduced libido. It can also protect against the brittle bone disease, osteoporosis, and heart disease in later life.

HRT contains oestrogen but in much lower doses than the pill. HRT may aggravate high blood pressure in women who already have the condition but it has been found to be quite safe in those who have their blood pressure checked regularly. HRT will not adversely affect any blood pressure drugs.

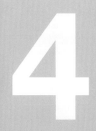

4

WHAT DOES IT MEAN?

WORD	DEFINITION
COMBINED ORAL CONTRACEPTIVE PILL	A contraceptive pill containing the two female sex hormones, oestrogen and progestogen.
HRT	Hormone replacement therapy, oestrogen and progestogen treatment, is prescribed at or after the menopause to counteract symptoms and protect against, or treat, brittle bones.
OESTROGEN	One of the two main female sex hormones. It is thought to be protective against heart disease before the menopause.
OSTEOPOROSIS	A disease in which the bones lose density, causing them to become brittle and break more easily. It is most common in women after the menopause.
PROGESTOGEN	One of the two major female sex hormones. The progestogen-only contraceptive pill may be less likely to cause a rise in blood pressure.

YOU REALLY NEED TO KNOW

◆ Some types of oral contraceptive pill cause a small rise in blood pressure.

◆ You are more likely to experience a rise in blood pressure if you are over 35, overweight, smoke or have previously had high blood pressure.

◆ HRT is less likely to cause a rise in blood pressure if your blood pressure is normal when you start using it.

◆ If you use the contraceptive pill or HRT your blood pressure should be checked regularly.

The pill and HRT

Medical conditions

Some medical conditions can increase the risk of high blood pressure; others make it inadvisable for certain types of blood-pressure-lowering drug to be prescribed.

Diabetes

There are two types of diabetes, a condition in which the the body is unable to use sugar (glucose) in the bloodstream either because the body does not produce enough insulin (type 1) or because it does not respond properly to what there is (type 2). Until recently the main treatment for diabetes has been to manage blood glucose levels through diet, drugs or injecting insulin. However, research shows that controlling blood pressure is just as important. One in every two people with type 2 diabetes (the most common) also has high blood pressure, putting them at unusually high risk of heart disease, stroke, blindness and, especially, kidney failure.

In someone with diabetes, the danger level of blood pressure is lower than the commonly accepted 140/85. For this reason, if you have diabetes your doctor will monitor you closely and may decide to treat you if your BP rises above 130/80.

Arthritis

Arthritis is inflammation causing pain, swelling and stiffness in the joints. There are many different types. Rheumatoid arthritis is a chronic condition which causes gradual destruction of the joints. It can also affect the heart, lungs and eyes. Arthritis is often treated with non-steroidal anti-inflammatory drugs (NSAIDs) which can increase blood pressure. If you have high blood pressure and arthritis your doctor will need to take into account both conditions when deciding how to treat you.

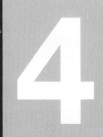

WHAT DOES IT MEAN?

CHRONIC CONDITION

A disease that goes on for a long time, such a diabetes, as opposed to one that can be treated and disappears.

INSULIN

A hormone produced by the pancreas which controls levels of glucose in the blood.

PANCREAS

One of the body's glands which produces the hormone insulin, needed to control blood glucose. Failure of the pancreas to produce enough insulin is a cause of diabetes.

Chest problems

People with asthma or other diseases causing breathing difficulties should not take beta-blocker drugs, so it is important to remind your doctor if you are being treated for such a condition. A minority of patients stop taking ACE inhibitors because they cause a dry irritating cough.

Heart disease

If you have angina (chest or arm pain caused by blocked arteries), beta blockers can help reduce the number of attacks you have. The doctor may prescribe other drugs such as those to lower cholesterol; this is also the case if you have had a heart attack as these drugs will reduce your chance of a further attack. ACE inhibitors and beta-blockers can be especially helpful as they can lower blood pressure as well as reducing the amount of work the heart has to do.

YOU REALLY NEED TO KNOW

◆ If you have diabetes it is especially important that your blood pressure and blood glucose levels are both controlled.

◆ If you have arthritis some drugs used to treat it may raise your blood pressure.

◆ It may be inadvisable for anyone with asthma or breathing problems to be prescribed beta blockers.

Medical conditions

Who should you tell?

Because of the implications for your health, there are a number of people who need to know if you are diagnosed with high blood pressure.

Medical practitioners

You should inform all your medical and paramedical practitioners, such as general or specialist doctors, physiotherapist, podiatrist or chiropodist, dentist, ambulance personnel and anyone else who treats you for a health-related problem.

It is important if you need treatment for any other condition because some drugs may interact with your blood-pressure-lowering drugs.

If you have to see another doctor, either in your GP's practice or in hospital , always make sure they know you are being treated for blood pressure.

If you are pregnant and have been diagnosed with high blood pressure you should inform your midwife and any other health professionals that you come into contact with, such as the obstetrician at the hospital.

Complementary practitioners

If you seek help from an alternative or complementary therapist such as a homeopath, acupuncturist, herbalist, aromatherapist or osteopath, tell them if you have high blood pressure. You should never stop taking any medication prescribed by your doctor on the advice of a complementary or alternative therapist.

Before accepting treatment from a complementary practitioner, check him or her out carefully. Ask about insurance, qualifications and accreditation from regulatory bodies. Steer clear of anyone who promises you a miracle cure. There isn't one.

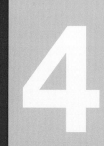

WHAT DOES IT MEAN?

AROMATHERAPY

A complementary therapy that uses essential oils from parts of plants and massage to restore wellbeing.

HERBALISM

A complementary therapy that uses herbs and herbal extracts to treat illness.

HOMEOPATHY

A therapy that involves treating illnesses with greatly diluted doses of the same substance that is thought to cause the illness.

OSTEOPATHY

A therapy that involves massage and manipulation of the bones to treat musculoskeletal pain, particularly of the back and limbs.

PARAMEDICAL

Health practitioners who support doctors, such as physiotherapists, podiatrists and ambulance personnel.

The pharmacist

Because certain high blood pressure treatments may interact with other types of medication it is important to tell the pharmacist you are being treated for high blood pressure. This applies whether you are getting a prescription medication or buying over-the-counter products for minor conditions. The pharmacist can be an invaluable source of advice on the possible interactions between one drug type and another.

YOU REALLY NEED TO KNOW

If you are diagnosed with high blood pressure and are being treated with drugs you should inform:

◆ All medical and paramedical practitioners with whom you come into contact.

◆ Your pharmacist.

◆ Your fitness instructor.

◆ Your insurance companies (personal and car).

You may also need to inform:

◆ Your employer.

◆ The driving licensing authority (the DVLA who issue your driving licence).

◆ Your holiday or tour operator.

Who should you tell?

Who should you tell?

Your employer

Raised blood pressure that's being treated will not usually be a problem at work. However, your employer may need to know about your condition if you have a job—such as roofing—that involves working at a height.

If you have high blood pressure you may not be allowed to join the police, fire service or armed services. If you already work in one of these jobs you may be allowed to continue working provided your blood pressure is controlled.

Driving licensing authority

The DVLA will not usually need to know if you have high blood pressure for an ordinary driving licence. However, if you drive a lorry, bus or other heavy vehicle special rules apply and you will need to inform them.

Whatever kind of licence you hold, you will need to inform the driving licensing authority if you have had a stroke or heart attack or if you have diabetes.

Insurance companies

If you are being treated for high blood pressure, you must inform any insurance company with whom you hold a health or life insurance policy—if you do not the policy may not be valid and when you come to make a claim there may not be a payment.

Also inform your insurance company of any changes in your medical state if you hold certain other types of policy which have a life assurance element, such as a mortgage endowment, and may also be affected. You should also mention your condition when you take out any insurance policy that covers you for medical treatment—holiday insurance, for example. You may find

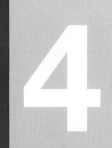

that some life insurance companies charge high premiums if you have high blood pressure. It is worth shopping around for the best policy.

Holidays and travel

Having high blood pressure should not prevent you going away on holiday. However, it pays to plan your trip carefully beforehand so you can be free from worries while you are away. As with many other medical conditions, when choosing your destination it is sensible to avoid very remote areas where it might be difficult to obtain medical attention, should you need it.

You may need to tell the tour operator and airline, especially if your high blood pressure is associated with another condition such as heart disease.

Allow yourself plenty of time to pack and prepare for your holiday to avoid undue stress and make sure that you allow plenty of time for the journey. If you are flying for longer than four hours take your daily aspirin just before you board the plane and drink plenty of water during the flight. Get up and walk around every two hours or so in order the prevent stagnation of the blood flow through the feet and legs.

Fitness instructors

If you belong to a gym or fitness club or embark on an activity such as an aerobics or yoga class you should inform the instructor that you have high blood pressure and whether you are taking medication for it.

This enables the instructor to make sure that you are not encouraged to do anything that could potentially exacerbate your condition, and ensures that you are insured while on the premises.

YOU REALLY NEED TO KNOW

◆ High blood pressure is not usually a problem at work, unless your job involves working at a height or driving a bus or lorry.

◆ You must inform the Driving Licensing Authority if you have had a stroke, a heart attack or have diabetes.

◆ Holiday insurance which precludes pre-existing conditions will not be valid if you are taking medication for raised blood pressure.

Who should you tell?

Understanding the jargon

Medicine is full of technical terms and words that can make a condition such as high blood pressure seem more daunting than it really is. Knowing what the terms mean can clarify your condition and enable you to communicate more easily with your doctor.

ACUTE—Used to describe a medical condition which comes on suddenly and lasts for only a limited period of time.

ANTIHYPERTENSIVE MEDICATION—Range of drugs administered to lower high blood pressure.

AORTA—The body's main artery, which leads from the heart, running down the back of the heart to the abdomen.

ARTERIES—The largest blood vessels in the body; they transport oxygen-rich blood from the heart to the rest of the body.

ARTERIOLES—Blood vessels which branch off the arteries and supply the organs and tissues with blood. Arterioles are smaller than arteries.

ATHEROSCLEROSIS—A disease in which the lining of the artery walls becomes furred with fatty deposits (such as cholesterol) plus decaying cells and other waste substances.

ARTERIOSCLEROSIS—A disease in which the artery walls become hard and thickened, and lose elasticity. It is commonly called hardening of the arteries.

CARDIOVASCULAR DISEASE—Disease affecting the heart and the blood vessels.

CHRONIC—A disease or medical condition which lasts for a long time.

CIRCULATORY SYSTEM—The heart and the blood vessels which are responsible for keeping blood flowing around the body.

DIASTOLE—The part of the heartbeat when the heart is at rest.

HYPERTENSION—High blood pressure.

HYPOTENSION—Low blood pressure.

ISCHAEMIA—Insufficient blood supply to an organ or tissue, usually caused by narrowing of the arteries.

PRE-ECLAMPSIA—A disease of the placenta causing high blood pressure during late pregnancy.

SPHYGNOMANOMETER—A device used to measure blood pressure, consisting of a cuff, pressure device, and a mercury column in a glass tube from which the measurements are read.

SYSTOLE—The part of the heartbeat when the heart is contracting.

THROMBUS—An abnormal blood clot.

VASCULAR—To do with the body's blood vessels.

VEINS—Blood vessels which return deoxygenated blood to the heart.

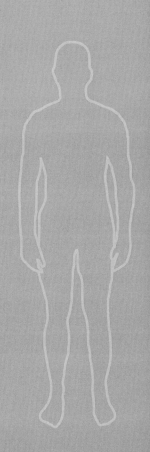

Useful addresses

WHERE TO GO FOR HELP

**ASH (ACTION ON SMOKING
AND HEALTH)**
102-108 Clifton Street
London EC2A 4HW
Tel: 0207 739 5902
www.ash.org.uk

For personal help to stop smoking
contact QUIT, a charity funded by the
Health Education Authority.
QUITline: 0800 002200
Asian QUITlines:
Bengali (Mondays) 0800 002244
Gujarati (Tuesdays) 0800 002255
Hindi (Wednesdays) 0800 002266
Punjabi (Thursdays) 0800 002277
Urdu (Fridays) 0800 002288

**BRITISH DIABETIC ASSOCIATION
(DIABETES UK)**
10 Queen Anne Street
London W1M OBD
Tel: 0207 323 1531
Careline: 0207 636 6112
www.diabetes.org.uk

BRITISH HEART FOUNDATION
14 Fitzhardinge Street
London W1H 4DH
Tel: 0207 935 0185
Information line: 0870 600 6566
www.bhf.org.uk

STROKE ASSOCIATION
Stroke House
Whitecross Street
London ECIY 8JJ
Tel: 0207 566 0300
www.stroke.org.uk

**INSTITUTE FOR COMPLEMENTARY
MEDICINE**
PO Box 194
London SE16 1QZ
Tel: 0207 237 5165 (answerphone)

Index

Index

Acknowledgements

Photographs: Simon Fraser/SPL, p.8–9, p43;
Saturn Stills/SPL, p.15, p.19; Eamon Mcnulty/SPL, p.30–31;
Light Productions/SPL, p.47; Jerome Yeats/SPL, p.48–49; Sam Ogden/SPL, p.56;
Andrew Sydenham, p.58; Laura Wickenden, p.60;
Faye Norman/SPL, p.62–63; Damien Lovegrove/SPL, p.73

Illustrations: Kuo Kang Chen, p.14, 24, 28; Martin Laurie, p.10, p.22, p.50, p.55